T0132380

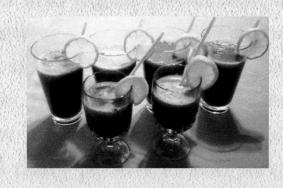

YOU Are What YOU Drink

Bernice Pinnock

To order additional copies of this book, contact:
Xlibris
844-714-8691
www.Xlibris.com
Orders@Xlibris.com

ISBN: Softcover   978-1-6698-6000-6
        EBook   978-1-6698-6001-3

Print information available on the last page

Rev. date: 03/30/2023

I dedicate this book to my late brother. He taught me how to hang in there during the most challenging times. My two children who love and support have given me the will to persevere. Lastly, to my cousin whose words of encouragement had inspired me to seek a college degree in history and that inspiration had prepared me for a journey in writing.

Contents

AUTHOR'S NOTES

I've been studying fruits and vegetables for over thirty years. When I got pregnant with my first child in 1983, I decided to do some research on health. I read nutritional books about calories, carbohydrates, cholesterol, and vitamins, to name a few. As I continued my research, I started experimenting with fresh fruits and vegetables by blending them together. To my surprise, they tasted great. Plus, I noticed how my skin was starting to develop a different kind of glow—not a pregnancy glow but a healthy glow—and the blended drinks gave me more energy. Also, I noticed how I was able to maintain healthy blood cholesterol, blood pressure, and weight. While people around me were getting sick with high cholesterol, high blood pressure, heart disease, diabetes, cancer, Covid-19, flu, and respiratory syncytial virus, I never once visited the hospital for those issues. My experience with blended fruit and vegetable drinks has helped me to maintain good health, and I hope that it will help you too. After all, _YOU Are What YOU Drink_.

BIOGRAPHY

When I gave birth to my last child, in 1988, I was burned out. At that point, I was a full-time student and full-time mother, and I was holding down an almost full-time job. It wasn't long before I was forced to settle for three hours of sleep per day. My husband, children, extended family, and friends could not believe the amount of energy I had. At times, I could not believe it either.

When I graduated from college with a B average, I received a scholarship to continue my education. In my opinion, I could not have achieved this goal without the help of my blended drink recipes. Not only did it give me the energy I needed to keep up with my busy lifestyle, but they also helped me to maintain good health with my weight, blood pressure, and cholesterol, among other things.

In 1988, I weighed 126 pounds, and thirty-four years later, my weight is about the same. Amazingly, I can fit into the same clothes I was wearing thirty-four years ago. Some people may credit this to genes, but I'm the smallest one in my family, thanks to my blended fruit and vegetable recipes.

I wrote this book to help those who don't enjoy eating vegetables and who want to get healthy. Personally, I struggled to eat certain vegetables too I didn't enjoy the way they tasted. Therefore, I had to find a way to consume vegetables without having to taste them. I tried juicing, but I noticed that there were more nutrients left behind in the strainer than in my glass. That was when I came up with the idea to ingest the best nutrient that I possibly could without getting the vegetable taste. Now, after thirty years of research and perfecting my recipes, I have discovered that you *can* enjoy the benefits and nutrition of vegetables without the taste. To ensure good health, it is essential to know what we are consuming. That is why my book contains a list of the beneficial factors of each blended recipe which makes one gallon. During my research, I discovered that it only takes fifteen minutes per day to help sustain a healthy lifestyle.

In 2010 Doctor Kenneth W. Harris, MD backed this book by giving me a letter. Twelve years later, my cholesterol level, glucose level, blood pressure and weight are still well maintained, and I contribute this to my fruit and vegetable blended drinks.

KENNETH W. HARRIS, MD
METRO MEMPHIS MEDICAL SPECIALISTS, INC.

February 18, 2010

Ms. Bernice Pinnock is a patient of mine and her physical health is exceptionally outstanding. Her cholesterol level, glucose level, blood pressure and weight are well maintained. It was pleasantly surprise to see a person of her age has a cholesterol level as low as a young adult. In my professional opinion I find that her healthy diet has a lot to do with her well being. I have personally studied research on fruits and vegetables. The research I have studied showed how the lack of fruits and vegetables may now be associated with certain forms of cancer. Therefore, in my professional opinion there is correlation between ones diet and ones health.

Kenneth W. Harris, MD

INTRODUCTION

With a trifecta of illnesses like a respiratory syncytial virus, COVID-19, and the flu, one thing should be on our mind and that is how to increase our immune function. We always hear that fresh fruits and vegetables are good for us, but what exactly is their impact when it comes to good health? Many studies have shown that incorporating fresh fruits and vegetables into our daily diet may help us achieve a healthier lifestyle. Fruit contains antioxidants that combat the destructive forces of free radicals and these may lead to oxidative stress, which some studies have shown can result in the premature aging of cells. Vegetables provide nutrients, minerals, phytochemicals, potassium, and fiber, among other important vitamins that are needed for good health. Consuming a balanced number of fresh fruits and vegetables every day may not only slow the signs of aging inside the body, but it may have a significant impact on the skin's appearance on the outside. According to Google, "A high-fiber plant-rich diet with plenty of fruits, vegetables, whole grains, and legumes appear to support the growth and maintenance of the beneficial microbes. *Certain helpful microbes break down fibers into short chain fatty acids, which have been shown to stimulate immune cell activity.*" According to research, a healthy immune system "can defeat invading disease-causing germs, such as bacteria, viruses, parasites" and can help fight against certain forms of cancer "while protecting healthy tissue." Also, a healthy immune system can reduce the risk of heart disease and stroke and lower the risk of eye and digestive problems. In writing this book I want to contribute my research to the Webster Dictionary, Encyclopedia, Google, and the many studies I have read on health throughout the years. In this book, I have included a very important list of fresh fruits and vegetables and their vitamin content that promote good health. Furthermore, I have provided thirty-five recipes for fresh fruit and vegetable blended drinks and their beneficial health benefits. This information is the result of my belief that we all have an obligation to educate one another on how to live a healthier lifestyle.

BENEFITS OF FRESH FRUIT AND VEGETABLE BLENDED DRINKS

There are excellent benefits of consuming fresh fruit and vegetable drinks. Not only does the combination strengthen the immune system to help fight cell-damaging free radicals in the body, which may lead to oxidative stress (studies show that this contributes to premature aging), but these foods contain an array of vitamins, minerals, fiber, as well as phytochemicals, plants compounds, and pigments that contain antioxidants. Some research has shown that antioxidant properties can help keep cells healthy and may help reduce LDL which is (*bad* cholesterol) levels while boosting HDL (*good* cholesterol) levels. A reduction in cholesterol levels may impede the development of certain forms of cancer and heart disease.

Today, we live in a society that has countless fast-food restaurants, and most of us have busy schedules. We tend to eat out frequently and we don't take the time to evaluate the food we eat. Many of us tend to overconsume meat, sugar, dairy products, and highly processed foods, the result of which tends to be an underconsumption of fruits and vegetables, which contain protective properties that may ward off certain diseases. It has been evinced through research that, for example, heart disease, cancer, hypertension, obesity, adult-onset diabetes, cirrhosis of the liver, and colon disease may be associated with the *standard American diet*. Therefore, I believe that one way to improve the *standard American diet* is to decrease the consumption of meat and dairy products and increase the consumption of fresh fruits and vegetables. One highly nutritious way to consume more fresh fruits and vegetables is in the form of a blended drink. Remember, we cannot maintain a healthy lifestyle without fresh fruits and vegetables which are full of nutrients, low in calories, and completely devoid of the saturated fats that may contribute to the development of heart disease.

Blended drinks composed of fresh fruits and vegetables are an excellent source of vitamins and minerals. For example, citrus fruits are high in cryptoxanthin—a pigment that may inhibit the growth of certain tumors—and also contain limonene compounds, which are thought to neutralize some cancer-causing chemicals. Specifically, research has shown that grapefruit and other pink fruits contain lycopene, which is a carotenoid pigment that may help combat certain forms of cancer.

Fresh fruit and vegetable blended drinks are highly nutritious, unlike processed fruit juices which are high in sugar, and depending on the drink, can also contain high levels of sodium. Furthermore, I believe that to receive the complete benefit of fruits and vegetables, it is better to eat or drink them when they are fresh. Studies have also shown that when cooked, some vegetables may lose their nutritional value; steamed vegetables may be over-steamed, leaving the nutritional value in the water instead of in the vegetable, and baked vegetables may be overbaked, evaporating the nutrients. On the other hand, fresh fruit and vegetable blended drinks have enormous benefits and are essential to maintaining a healthy lifestyle. The American Institute for Cancer Research has suggested that a meal should be composed of at least two-thirds plant-based foods like vegetables, fruits, whole grains, and beans, and no more than one-third animal protein.

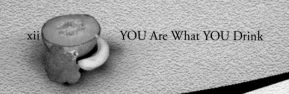

VITAMIN CATALOG

Research shows:

<u>Vitamin A</u> is one of the few vitamins that can be absorbed through the skin. The nourishing benefits of vitamin A is that it helps to keep the skin soft and young looking.

(Vitamin A may help maintain the eyes, skin, bones, teeth, and a healthy immune system.)

<u>Vitamin B</u> plays an important role in energy metabolism in the body. Vitamin B-12 is essential for the normal formation of healthy red blood cells, and it contributes to the health of the nervous system. Vitamins B-12 and B-6 support heart health. Vitamin B-12 is found in animal products like liver and shellfish.

<u>Vitamin C</u> supports immune function. As an antioxidant, it helps neutralize harmful free radicals in cells. Vitamin C helps the body to maintain strong teeth, gums, bones, and muscles. Also, it helps to ward off colds.

(Research has shown that vitamin C may help reduce the risk of certain forms of cancer.)

<u>Vitamin D</u> assists the body's calcium to maintain strong bones, and it plays an important role in the immune system.

(Vitamin D is essential to reduce osteoporosis in the elderly. It is also important for good health.)

<u>Vitamin D</u> contains the formation of prothrombin which is necessary for normal blood clotting.

<u>Vitamin E</u> is an antioxidant which means it helps fight the destructive forces of free radicals with our natural antioxidant formulas.

(Vitamin E may help with healthy aging.)

<u>Iron</u> helps aid a healthy blood supply which is full of oxygen.

(Iron may help with healthy blood flow.)

<u>Vitamin K</u> is also a companion to calcium and vitamin D.

NUTRITION CATALOG

Research shows:

<u>Beta-carotene</u> is an immune system enhancer and antioxidant. It helps fight cells that are damaging free radicals in the body, and free radicals can lead to oxidative stress. Studies have shown oxidative stress contributes to aging.

(Beta-carotene may help with healthy aging.)

<u>Lutein and Zeaxanthin</u> are two carotenoids which may help protect against age-related eye disorders.

<u>Lycopene</u> is an antioxidant, and it helps convert beta-carotene into vitamin A, which helps give, sharp night vision, and smooth skin.

<u>Omega-3 Fatty Acids</u> may help protect the heart. Also, may help reduce the risk of a stroke, lower cholesterol levels, and alleviate arthritis.

<u>Potassium</u> helps keep blood pressure down and it aids muscle contractions. It helps maintain healthy electrical activity in the heart and rapid transmission of nerve impulses throughout the body.

(Potassium may help aid a healthy heart.)

<u>Proanthocyanidins</u> may work as antioxidants and block nitrosamines from forming and may protect the heart and cardiovascular system.

<u>Phytonutrients/Phytochemicals</u> may help reduce the risk of diseases from aging, such as Alzheimer's, osteoporosis, cancer, and heart disease.

I have mentioned a few of the essential vitamins and minerals your body needs to maintain good health. The few I listed pertain to the fruit and vegetable blended recipes in this book.

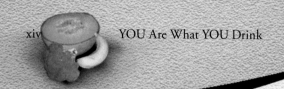

FRUIT CATALOG

<u>Research shows:</u>

<u>Apples</u> are a good source of pectin, a soluble fiber that may help reduce the risk of blood cholesterol, and a good source of vitamin C.

<u>Apricot</u> is high in vitamin A and contains potassium.

<u>Bananas</u> are high in Vitamin B6 and a good source of vitamin C, fiber, and potassium.

<u>Berries (Blueberries)</u> are high in fiber, antioxidants, phytochemicals, and vitamins, and a potent source of vitamin C.

<u>Cantaloupe</u> is high in vitamin C and a good source of vitamins B6 and A.

<u>Grapefruit</u> is high in vitamin C and contains antioxidants that may help reduce the risk of certain forms of cancer.

<u>Grapes</u> contain phytochemicals that may reduce the risk of heart disease, and it has the beneficial substance found in red wine.

<u>Honeydew</u> is high in vitamin C and a good source of potassium.

<u>Lemons</u> are high in vitamin C and fiber, and they contain bioflavonoid that may help reduce the risk of certain forms of cancer.

<u>Nectarine</u> is high in vitamin A, a good source of vitamin C, and contains phytochemicals that promote good health.

<u>Oranges</u> are high in vitamin C, a good source of folate, fiber, and contain antioxidants that promote good health.

<u>Papaya</u> is high in vitamin C.

<u>Peaches</u> are a good source of vitamin A and C.

<u>Pears</u> are a good source of dietary fiber and vitamin C.

<u>Pineapples</u> are high in vitamin C.

<u>Plums</u> are a good source of vitamin C.

<u>Strawberries</u> are a good source of vitamin C and potassium.

<u>Watermelon</u> is high in vitamin C, a good source of lycopene, and an antioxidant that may help protect against certain forms of cancer.

Information Purposes:

<u>Kiwi</u> is high in vitamin C and a good source of fiber.

<u>Mango</u> is high in vitamin A, and C.

VEGETABLE CATALOG

Research shows:

<u>Broccoli</u> is high in vitamin A and C and is a cruciferous vegetable that contains phytochemicals, which may help reduce the risk of certain forms of cancer.

<u>Cabbage</u> is high in vitamin C and is a cruciferous vegetable that contains phytochemicals, which may help reduce the risk of certain forms of cancer.

<u>Carrot</u> is high in vitamin A (beta-carotene), a good source of

fiber, and contains phytochemicals, which may help reduce the risk of certain forms of cancer and heart disease.

<u>Collard greens</u> are high in vitamin A (beta-carotene), vitamin C, and folate, and are a good source of fiber and calcium. It is a cruciferous vegetable that contains phytochemicals that may help reduce the risk of certain forms of cancer.

<u>Kale</u> contains vitamin A, antioxidants, minerals, and potent phytochemicals.

<u>Lettuce</u> (Romaine) can be a good source of folate, next to eight times vitamin A and six times vitamin C than (iceberg) lettuce.

<u>Mustard greens</u> are loaded with vitamins and minerals and and are high in vitamin A and C and iron.

<u>Spinach</u> contains vitamin A (beta-carotene) and is a good source of vitamin C and minerals.

<u>Squash</u> is high in vitamins A and C, magnesium, and potassium.

<u>Tomatoes</u> are high in vitamin C, a good source of vitamin A,

phosphorus, potassium, and contain antioxidants and lycopene.

<u>Turnip greens</u> are an excellent source of vitamin A and B.

BEST TO GO ORGANIC

When selecting fresh fruits and vegetables to blend, it is best to go organic. Organic products are grown without the use of chemical additives; this means they contain a lower level of pesticide residue than standard commercial produce. Research states that "the quality of fruits and vegetables is only as good as the soil they come from." If you choose to purchase non-organic produce, there are all-natural solutions on the market that help remove the leftover wax, chemicals, and soil residue from these products that cannot be washed off by ordinary tap water. Hence, before blending, always remember to wash all fruits and vegetables thoroughly.

Adding sugar to blended drink recipes is not recommended. However, if you choose to include sugar, try to go organic. For example, brown sugar composed of organic sugar cane contains some nutritional value, i.e., it has 2 percent vitamin C and 11 percent iron, and plain white and brown sugars do not.

BUYING EQUIPMENT

When buying equipment, purchase a five-, six-, or seven-cup blender with a minimum power output of 450 watts. The wattage is the horsepower of a blender and this controls how fast the blender blends; thus, the wattage may affect the quality of the liquid produced by the blender. The ideal blender is clear glass with a liquefy setting. The glass makes it easier to see the fresh fruits and vegetables while they are blending, and the use of the liquefy setting ensures that the fruits and vegetables blend faster. It is also advisable to purchase a clear two-inch measuring cup, as it provides clearly visible measurements. Moreover, purchase a clear plastic one-gallon container; this allows you to see the mixture while you shake well before serving. Other items to purchase are a measuring tape, a cutting board, a knife, and a timer. You can also purchase a blender with a built-in timer; however, if you do not purchase this type of blender, just time it to five minutes.

FRESH FRUIT AND VEGETABLE BLENDED COMBINATIONS

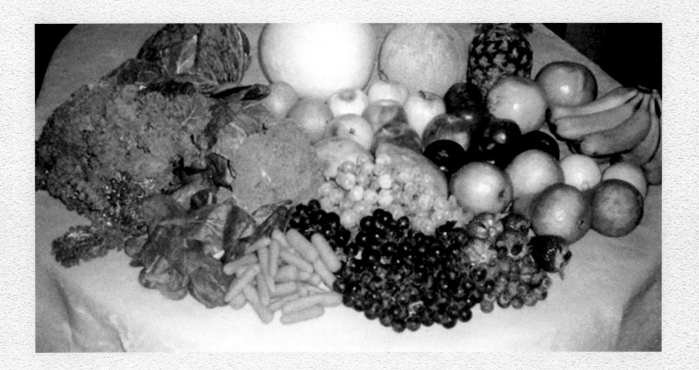

When blending fresh fruits and vegetables, the water measurement for blending and time blending may vary from the recommended time in the recipes. It all depends upon the cup size of the blender purchased.

MIDMORNING BLEND

2 peaches
2 oranges (seedless)
½ cantaloupe
20 baby carrots
3 kale leaves
8 cups of water
(Remember to wash all fruits and vegetables thoroughly.)

1. Cut two peaches into four pieces each and remove the seeds. Peel two seedless oranges and cut them into four pieces each. Remove twenty baby carrots from the bag. Cut the stems off three kale leaves and cut each leaf into three pieces. Take one cantaloupe and cut it in half, remove the skin, and cut it into eight pieces. Place the other portion of the cantaloupe in the refrigerator.

2. Place in a blender eight pieces of peaches, eight pieces of oranges, and twenty baby carrots, and add four to four and a half cups of water. Before blending, at the top of the blender, leave one to one and a half inches empty to leave room for blending. Blend or liquefy for five minutes. Place in the gallon container. (This may vary depending on the cup size of the blender.)

3. Place in the blender eight pieces of cantaloupe and nine pieces of kale leaves and add water. Before blending, at the top of the blender, leave one to one and a half inches empty to leave room for blending. Blend or liquefy for five minutes. Place in the gallon container. If needed, add additional water to the gallon to make eight cups of water. (This may vary depending on the cup size of the blender.)

4. Place the top on the gallon container and shake well for a few minutes. Adding sugar is not recommended, and if on a diet, avoid using sugar. To sweeten, add no more than one-third cup of organic whole cane sugar (brown sugar). Stir and place in refrigerator until cold. For a fresh taste, drink within three to five days or store in the freezer.

Research shows, over time, this may help maintain a healthy immune system.

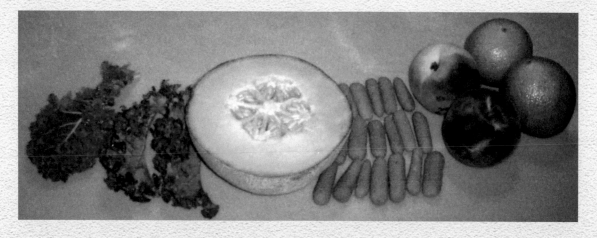

PINE BURST BLEND

2 oranges (seedless)
2 apples
1 papaya
2 plums
½ pineapple
3 kale leaves
8 cups of water
(Remember to wash all fruits and vegetables thoroughly.)

1. Cut two apples into four pieces each and remove the seeds. Peel two seedless oranges and cut them into four pieces each. Peel one papaya, remove the seeds, and cut it into four pieces. Cut two plums into four pieces each and remove the seeds. Cut the stems off three kale leaves and cut each leaf into three pieces. Take one pineapple and cut it in half. Remove the skin and crown and cut it into eight pieces. Place the other portion of the pineapple in the refrigerator.

2. Place in a blender eight pieces of apples, eight pieces of oranges, four pieces of papaya, and eight pieces of plums, and add four to four and a half cups of water. Before blending, at the top of the blender, leave one to one and a half inches empty to leave room for blending. Blend or liquefy for five minutes. Place in the gallon container. (This may vary depending on the cup size of the blender.)

3. Place in the blender eight pieces of pineapple and nine pieces of kale leaves and add water. Before blending, at the top of the blender, leave one to one and a half inches empty to leave room for blending. Blend or liquefy for five minutes. Place in the gallon container. If needed, add additional water to the gallon to make eight cups of water. (This may vary depending on the cup size of the blender.)

4. Place the top on the gallon container and shake well for a few minutes. Adding sugar is not recommended, and if on a diet, avoid using sugar. To sweeten, add no more than one-third cup of organic whole cane sugar (brown sugar). Stir and place in refrigerator until cold. For a fresh taste, drink within three to five days or store in the freezer.

Research shows, over time, this may help maintain a healthy immune system.

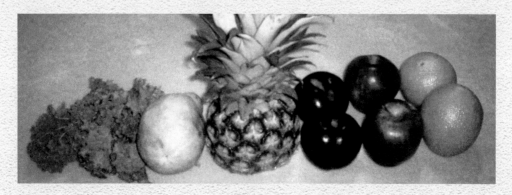

HONEY BURST BLEND

½ honeydew
2 oranges (seedless)
2 apples
3 tomatoes (Roma)
4 fresh cabbage leaves
7 cups of water
(Remember to wash all fruits and vegetables thoroughly.)

1. Cut two apples into four pieces each and remove the seeds. Peel two seedless oranges and cut them into four pieces each. Cut three Roma tomatoes into two pieces each. Break off four fresh cabbage leaves from a head of cabbage and cut each leaf into three pieces. Take one honeydew and cut it in half, remove the skin, and cut it into eight pieces. Place the other portion of cabbage and honeydew in the refrigerator.

2. Place in a blender eight pieces of apples, eight pieces of oranges, and eight pieces of honeydew, and add three to three and a half cups of water. Before blending, at the top of the blender, leave one to one and a half inches empty to leave room for blending. Blend or liquefy for five minutes. Place in the gallon container. (This may vary depending on the cup size of the blender.)

3. Place in the blender six pieces of Roma tomatoes and twelve pieces of cabbage leaves and add water. Before blending, at the top of the blender, leave one to one and a half inches empty to leave room for blending. Blend or liquefy for five minutes. Place in the gallon container. If needed, add additional water to the gallon to make seven cups of water. (This may vary depending on the cup size of the blender.)

4. Place the top on the gallon container and shake well for a few minutes. Adding sugar is not recommended, and if on a diet, avoid using sugar. To sweeten, add no more than one-third cup of organic whole cane sugar (brown sugar). Stir and place in refrigerator until cold. For a fresh taste, drink within three to five days or store in the freezer.

Research shows, over time, this may help reduce blood cholesterol and may help reduce the risk of certain forms of cancer and promote good health.

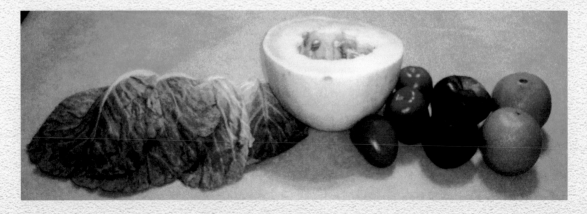

GOOD AND FRUITY BLEND

½ cantaloupe
2 bananas
2 oranges (seedless)
10 strawberries
20 baby carrots
20 baby spinach leaves
7 to 8 cups of water
(Remember to wash all fruits and vegetables thoroughly.)

1. Peel two seedless oranges and cut them into four pieces each. Peel two bananas and cut them into three pieces each. Remove the green leaves off the top of ten strawberries and cut each strawberry into two pieces. Remove twenty baby carrots from the bag, and remove twenty fresh baby spinach leaves from the bag. Take one cantaloupe and cut it in half, remove the skin, and cut it into eight pieces. Place the other portion of cantaloupe in the refrigerator.

2. Place in a blender six pieces of oranges, six pieces of bananas, and eight pieces of cantaloupe, and add three to three and a half cups of water. Before blending, at the top of the blender, leave one to one and a half inches empty to leave room for blending. Blend or liquefy for five minutes. Place in the gallon container. (This may vary depending on the cup size of the blender.)

3. Place in the blender two pieces of oranges, twenty pieces of strawberries, twenty baby carrots, and twenty baby spinach, and add water. Before blending, at the top of the blender, leave one to one and a half inches empty to leave room for blending. Blend or liquefy for five minutes. Place in the gallon container. If needed, add additional water to the gallon to make seven to eight cups of water. (This may vary depending on the cup size of the blender.)

4. Place the top on the gallon container and shake well for a few minutes. Adding sugar is not recommended, and if on a diet, avoid using sugar. To sweeten, add no more than one-third cup of organic whole cane sugar (brown sugar). Stir and place in refrigerator until cold. For a fresh taste, drink within three to five days or store in the freezer.

Research shows, over time, this may help promote good health.

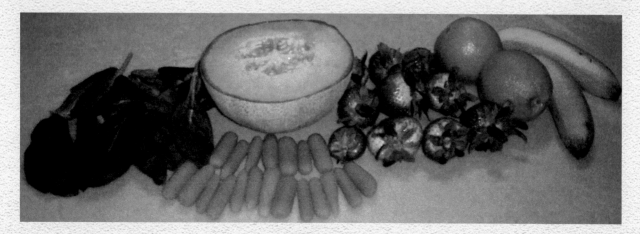

FRUITY BURST BLEND

2 pears
2 apples
2 oranges (seedless)
2 bananas
2 tomatoes (Roma)
1 broccoli bunch
8 cups of water
(Remember to wash all fruits and vegetables thoroughly.)

1. Cut two apples into four pieces each and remove the seeds. Peel two seedless oranges and cut them into four pieces each. Cut two pears into four pieces each and remove the stalk. Peel two bananas and cut them into three pieces each. Cut two Roma tomatoes into two pieces each. Take one broccoli bunch and cut off the stem and chop the leaves into pieces.

2. Place in a blender eight pieces of apples, eight pieces of oranges, and eight pieces of pears, and add four to four and a half cups of water. Before blending, at the top of the blender, leave one to one and a half inches empty to leave room for blending. Blend or liquefy for five minutes. Place in the gallon container. (This may vary depending on the cup size of the blender).

3. Place in the blender six pieces of bananas, four pieces of Roma tomatoes, and broccoli leaves, and add water. Before blending, at the top of the blender, leave one to one and a half inches empty to leave room for blending. Blend or liquefy for five minutes. Place in the gallon container. If needed, add additional water to the gallon to make eight cups of water. (This may vary depending on the cup size of the blender.)

4. Place the top on the gallon container and shake well for a few minutes. Adding sugar is not recommended, and if on a diet, avoid using sugar. To sweeten, add no more than one-third cup of organic whole cane sugar (brown sugar). Stir and place in refrigerator until cold. For a fresh taste, drink within three to five days or store in the freezer.

Research shows this contains antioxidants that promote good health.

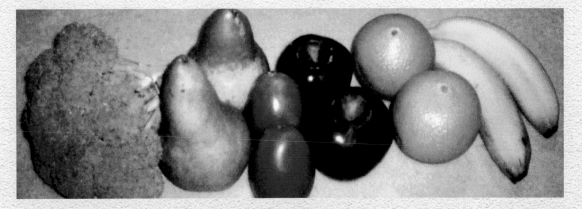

APPLE FRUITY BLEND

5 apples
3 tomatoes (Roma)
2 bananas
3 mustard greens (leaves)
20 baby carrots
9 cups of water
(Remember to wash all fruits and vegetables thoroughly.)

1. Cut five apples into four pieces each and remove the seeds. Peel two bananas and cut them into three pieces each. Cut three Roma tomatoes into two pieces each, remove twenty baby carrots from the bag, and cut three mustard leaves into three pieces each leaf.

2. Place in a blender twelve pieces of apples, six pieces of Roma tomatoes, and six pieces of bananas, and add three and a half to four cups of water. Before blending, at the top of the blender, leave one to one and a half inches empty to leave room for blending. Blend or liquefy for five minutes. Place in the gallon container. (This may vary depending on the cup size of the blender.)

3. Place in the blender eight pieces of apples, twenty baby carrots, and nine pieces of mustard leaves, and add water. Before blending, at the top of the blender, leave one to one and a half inches empty to leave room for blending. Blend or liquefy for five minutes. Place in the gallon container. If needed, add additional water to the gallon to make nine cups of water. (This may vary depending on the cup size of the blender.)

4. Place the top on the gallon container and shake well for a few minutes. Adding sugar is not recommended, and if on a diet, avoid using sugar. To sweeten, add no more than one-third cup of organic whole cane sugar (brown sugar). Stir and place in refrigerator until cold. For a fresh taste, drink within three to five days or store in the freezer.

Research shows, over time, this may help reduce blood cholesterol and promote good health.

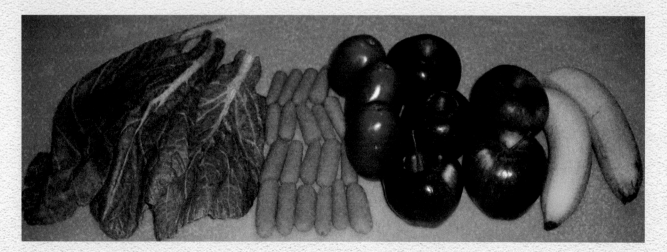

MUSTARD BLEND

4 apples
4 oranges (seedless)
2 tomatoes (Roma)
15 baby carrots
4 mustard greens (leaves)
10 cups of water
(Remember to wash all fruits and vegetables thoroughly.)

1. Cut four apples into four pieces each and remove the seeds. Peel four seedless oranges and cut them into four pieces each, cut two Roma tomatoes into two pieces each, remove fifteen baby carrots from the bag, and cut four mustard leaves into three pieces each.

2. Place in a blender twelve pieces of apples, twelve pieces of oranges, and four pieces of Roma tomatoes, and add three and a half to four cups of water. Before blending, at the top of the blender, leave one to one and a half inches empty to leave room for blending. Blend or liquefy for five minutes. Place in the gallon container. (This may vary depending on the cup size of the blender.)

3. Place in the blender fifteen baby carrots, twelve pieces of mustard leaves, four pieces of oranges, and four pieces of apples, and add water. Before blending, at the top of the blender, leave one to one and a half inches empty to leave room for blending. Blend or liquefy for five minutes. Place in the gallon container. If needed, add additional water to the gallon to make ten cups of water. (This may vary depending on the cup size of the blender).

4. Place the top on the gallon container and shake well for a few minutes. Adding sugar is not recommended, and if on a diet, avoid using sugar. To sweeten, add no more than one-third cup of organic whole cane sugar (brown sugar). Stir and place in refrigerator until cold. For a fresh taste, drink within three to five days or store in the freezer.

Research shows, over time, this may support the immune system and support good health.

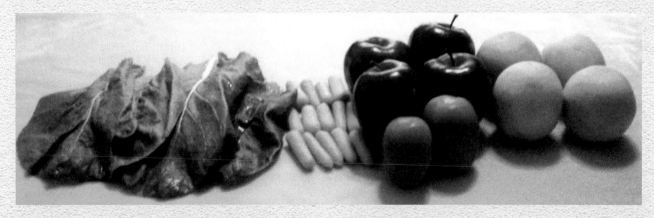

JOYFUL BLEND

2 apples
2 oranges (seedless)
3 bananas
1 lemon
20 baby carrots
2 tomatoes (Roma)
1 broccoli bunch
9 cups of water
(Remember to wash all fruits and vegetables thoroughly.)

1. Cut two apples into four pieces each and remove the seeds. Peel two seedless oranges and cut them into four pieces each. Peel three bananas and cut them into three pieces each. Peel one lemon and cut it into two pieces, cut two Roma tomatoes into two pieces each, and remove twenty baby carrots from the bag. Take one broccoli bunch and cut off the stem and chop the leaves into pieces.

2. Place in a blender eight pieces of apples, eight pieces of oranges, two pieces of lemons, and three pieces of bananas add four to four and a half cups of water. Before blending, at the top of the blender, leave one to one and a half inches empty to leave room for blending. Blend or liquefy for five minutes. Place in the gallon container. (This may vary depending on the cup size of the blender.)

3. Place in the blender six pieces of bananas, four pieces of Roma tomatoes, twenty baby carrots, and broccoli leaves, and add water. Before blending, at the top of the blender, leave one to one and a half inches empty to leave room for blending. Blend or liquefy for five minutes. Place in the gallon container. If needed, add additional water to the gallon to make nine cups of water. (This may vary depending on the cup size of the blender.)

4. Place the top on the gallon container and shake well for a few minutes. Adding sugar is not recommended, and if on a diet, avoid using sugar. To sweeten, add no more than one-third cup of organic whole cane sugar (brown sugar). Stir and place in refrigerator until cold. For a fresh taste, drink within three to five days or store in the freezer.

Research shows, over time, this may help reduce the risk of certain forms of cancer and heart disease and promote good health.

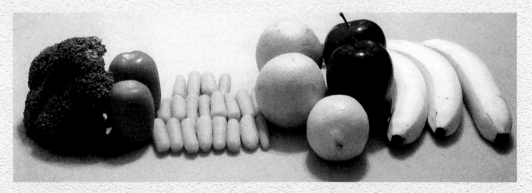

CANTA-DEW BLEND

½ honey dew
½ cantaloupe
2 oranges (seedless)
20 baby carrots
1 kale leaf
7 ½ cups of water
(Remember to wash all fruits and vegetables thoroughly.)

1. Peel two seedless oranges and cut them into four pieces each, cut the stem off one kale leaf and cut it into three pieces, and remove twenty baby carrots from the bag. Take one cantaloupe and cut it in half, remove the skin, and cut it into eight pieces. Place the other portion of cantaloupe in the refrigerator. Take one honeydew and cut it in half, remove the skin, and cut it into eight pieces. Place the other portion of honeydew in the refrigerator.

2. Place in a blender four pieces of oranges, sixteen baby carrots, and eight pieces of cantaloupe, and add three to three and a half cups of water. Before blending, at the top of the blender, leave one to one and a half inches empty to leave room for blending. Blend or liquefy for five minutes. Place in the gallon container. (This may vary depending on the cup size of the blender.)

3. Place in the blender four pieces of oranges, four baby carrots, three pieces of kale leaves, and eight pieces of honeydew, and add water. Before blending, at the top of the blender, leave one to one and a half inches empty to leave room for blending. Blend or liquefy for five minutes. Place in the gallon container. If needed, add additional water to the gallon to make seven and a half cups of water. (This may vary depending on the cup size of the blender.)

4. Place the top on the gallon container and shake well for a few minutes. Adding sugar is not recommended, and if on a diet, avoid using sugar. To sweeten, add no more than one-third cup of organic whole cane sugar (brown sugar). Stir and place in refrigerator until cold. For a fresh taste, drink within three to five days or store in the freezer.

Research shows, over time, this may help reduce the risk of certain forms of cancer and heart disease and promote good health.

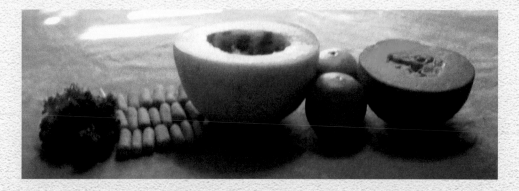

SUNRISE BLEND

½ cantaloupe
10 strawberries
2 bananas
4 cabbage leaves
10 baby spinach leaves
8 cups of water
(Remember to wash all fruits and vegetables thoroughly.)

1. Peel two bananas and cut them into three pieces each. Remove the green leaves off the top of ten strawberries and cut each strawberry into two pieces. Remove ten fresh baby spinach leaves from the bag. Break off four fresh cabbage leaves from a head of cabbage and cut each leaf into three pieces. Take one cantaloupe and cut it in half, remove the skin, and cut it into eight pieces. Place the other portion of cabbage and cantaloupe in the refrigerator.

2. Place in a blender twenty pieces of strawberries and eight pieces of cantaloupe and add three and a half to four cups of water. Before blending, at the top of the blender, leave one to one and a half inches empty to leave room for blending. Blend or liquefy for five minutes. Place in the gallon container. (This may vary depending on the cup size of the blender.)

3. Place in the blender ten baby spinach leaves, six pieces of bananas, and twelve pieces of cabbage leaves, and add water. Before blending, at the top of the blender, leave one to one and a half inches empty to leave room for blending. Blend or liquefy for five minutes. Place in the gallon container. If needed, add additional water to the gallon to make eight cups of water. (This may vary depending on the cup size of the blender.)

4. Place the top on the gallon container and shake well for a few minutes. Adding sugar is not recommended, and if on a diet, avoid using sugar. To sweeten, add no more than one-third cup of organic whole cane sugar (brown sugar). Stir and place in refrigerator until cold. For a fresh taste, drink within three to five days or store in the freezer.

Research shows, over time, this may help reduce the risk of certain forms of cancer and may help support the immune system.

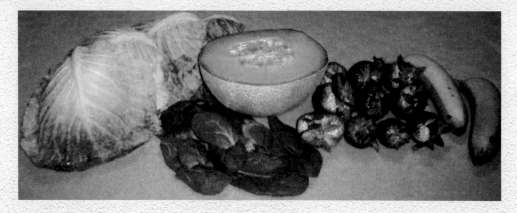

CANTA-PLUS BLEND

½ cantaloupe
2 apples
2 pears
2 tomatoes (Roma)
20 baby spinach leaves
6 to 7 cups of water
(Remember to wash all fruits and vegetables thoroughly.)

1. Cut two apples into four pieces each and remove the seeds. Cut two pears into four pieces each and remove the stalk. Cut two Roma tomatoes into two pieces each. Remove twenty fresh baby spinach leaves from the bag. Take one cantaloupe and cut it in half, remove the skin, and cut it into eight pieces. Place the other portion of cantaloupe in the refrigerator.

2. Place in a blender twenty baby spinach leaves and eight pieces of cantaloupe and add two and a half to three cups of water. Before blending, at the top of the blender, leave one to one and a half inches empty to leave room for blending. Blend or liquefy for five minutes. Place in the gallon container. (This may vary depending on the cup size of the blender.)

3. Place in the blender eight pieces of apples, eight pieces of pears, and four pieces of Roma tomatoes, and add water. Before blending, at the top of the blender, leave one to one and a half inches empty to leave room for blending. Blend or liquefy for five minutes. Place in the gallon container. If needed, add additional water to the gallon to make six to seven cups of water. (This may vary depending on the cup size of the blender.)

4. Place the top on the gallon container and shake well for a few minutes. Adding sugar is not recommended, and if on a diet, avoid using sugar. To sweeten, add no more than one-third cup of organic whole cane sugar (brown sugar). Stir and place in refrigerator until cold. For a fresh taste, drink within three to five days or store in the freezer.

Research shows, over time, this may help reduce blood cholesterol and help support the immune system.

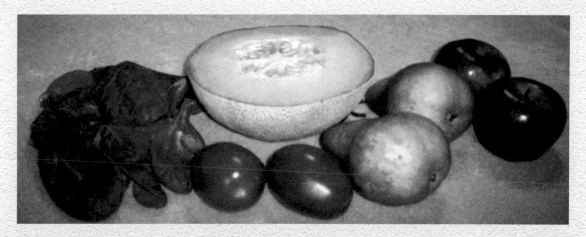

STRAWBERRY BLEND

25 strawberries
2 oranges (seedless)
2 apples
3 tomatoes (Roma)
20 baby spinach leaves
8 ½ cups of water
(Remember to wash all fruits and vegetables thoroughly.)

1. Cut two apples into four pieces each and remove the seeds. Peel two seedless oranges and cut them into four pieces each. Cut three Roma tomatoes into two pieces each. Remove the green leaves off the top of twenty-five strawberries and cut each strawberry into two pieces. Remove twenty fresh baby spinach leaves from the bag.

2. Place in a blender fifty pieces of strawberries and eight pieces of apples and add four to four and a half cups of water. Before blending, at the top of the blender, leave one to one and a half inches empty to leave room for blending. Blend or liquefy for five minutes. Place in the gallon container. (This may vary depending on the cup size of the blender.)

3. Place in the blender twenty baby spinach leaves, eight pieces of oranges, and six pieces of Roma tomatoes, and add water. Before blending, at the top of the blender, leave one to one and a half inches empty to leave room for blending. Blend or liquefy for five minutes. Place in the gallon container. If needed, add additional water to the gallon to make eight and a half cups of water. (This may vary depending on the cup size of the blender.)

4. Place the top on the gallon container and shake well for a few minutes. Adding sugar is not recommended, and if on a diet, avoid using sugar. To sweeten, add no more than one-third cup of organic whole cane sugar (brown sugar). Stir and place in refrigerator until cold. For a fresh taste, drink within three to five days or store in the freezer.

Research shows, over time, this may help reduce blood cholesterol and promote good health.

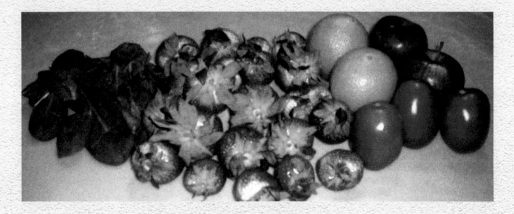

HONEY BLEND

½ honeydew
2 bananas
2 apples
2 tomatoes (Roma)
3 cabbage leaves
7 cups of water
(Remember to wash all fruits and vegetables thoroughly.)

1. Peel two bananas and cut them into three pieces each. Cut two apples into four pieces each and remove the seeds. Cut two Roma tomatoes into two pieces each. Break off three fresh cabbage leaves from a head of cabbage and cut each leaf into three pieces. Take one honeydew and cut it in half, remove the skin, and cut it into eight pieces. Place the other portion of cabbage and honeydew in the refrigerator.

2. Place in a blender eight pieces of honeydew and four pieces of cabbage and add two and a half to three cups of water. Before blending, at the top of the blender, leave one to one and a half inches empty to leave room for blending. Blend or liquefy for five minutes. Place in the gallon container. (This may vary depending on the cup size of the blender.)

3. Place in the blender six pieces of bananas, eight pieces of apples, four pieces of Roma tomatoes, and five pieces of cabbage leaves, and add water. Before blending, at the top of the blender, leave one to one and a half inches empty to leave room for blending. Blend or liquefy for five minutes. Place in the gallon container. If needed, add additional water to the gallon to make seven cups of water. (This may vary depending on the cup size of the blender.)

4. Place the top on the gallon container and shake well for a few minutes. Adding sugar is not recommended, and if on a diet, avoid using sugar. To sweeten, add no more than one-third cup of organic whole cane sugar (brown sugar). Stir and place in refrigerator until cold. For a fresh taste, drink within three to five days or store in the freezer.

Research shows, over time, this may help reduce the risk of certain forms of cancer and promote good health.

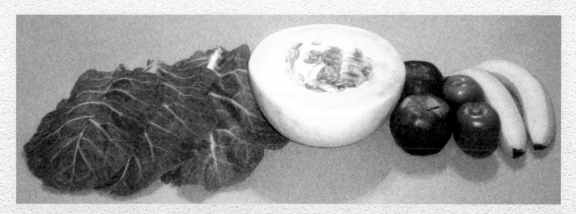

HONEY FRUIT BLEND

½ honeydew
2 bananas
2 oranges (seedless)
2 apples
20 baby carrots
1 broccoli bunch
7 ½ cups of water
(Remember to wash all fruits and vegetables thoroughly.)

1. Peel two bananas and cut them into three pieces each. Peel two seedless oranges and cut them into four pieces each. Cut two apples into four pieces each and remove the seeds. Remove twenty baby carrots from the bag. Take one broccoli bunch and cut off the stem and chop the leaves into pieces. Take one honeydew and cut them in half, remove the skin, and cut them into eight pieces. Place the other portion of honeydew in the refrigerator.

2. Place in a blender eight pieces of honeydew and add three to three and a half cups of water. Before blending, at the top of the blender, leave one to one and a half inches empty to leave room for blending. Blend or liquefy for five minutes. Place in the gallon container. (This may vary depending on the cup size of the blender.)

3. Place in the blender six pieces of bananas, four pieces of oranges, and four pieces of apples, and add water. Before blending, at the top of the blender, leave one to one and a half inches empty to leave room for blending. Blend or liquefy for five minutes. Place in the gallon container. (This may vary depending on the cup size of the blender.)

4. Place in the blender twenty baby carrots, four pieces of oranges, two pieces of apples, and broccoli leaves, and add water. Before blending, at the top of the blender, leave one to one and a half inches empty to leave room for blending. Blend or liquefy for five minutes. If needed, add additional water to the gallon to make seven and a half cups of water. (This may vary depending on the cup size of the blender.)

5. Place the top on the gallon container and shake well for a few minutes. Adding sugar is not recommended, and if on a diet, avoid using sugar. To sweeten, add no more than one-third cup of organic whole cane sugar (brown sugar). Stir and place in refrigerator until cold. For a fresh taste, drink within three to five days or store in the freezer.

Research shows, over time, this may help reduce the risk of certain forms of cancer and may help reduce blood cholesterol.

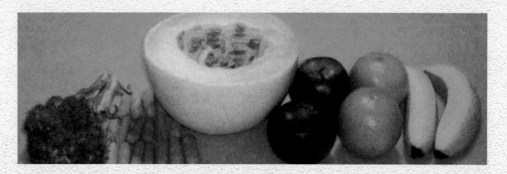

FRUITY BURST BLEND

3 bananas
2 apples
2 oranges (seedless)
3 tomatoes (Roma)
20 baby carrots
1 broccoli bunch
8 cups of water
(Remember to wash all fruits and vegetables thoroughly.)

1. Peel three bananas and cut them into three pieces each. Peel two seedless oranges and cut them into four pieces each. Cut two apples into four pieces each and remove the seeds. Cut three Roma tomatoes into two pieces each. Remove twenty baby carrots from the bag. Take one broccoli bunch and cut off the stem and chop the leaves into pieces.

2. Place in a blender nine pieces of bananas, eight pieces of apples, and two pieces of Roma tomato, and add three and a half to four cups of water. Before blending, at the top of the blender, leave one to one and a half empty to leave room for blending. Blend or liquefy for five minutes. Place in the gallon container. (This may vary depending on the cup size of the blender.)

3. Place in blender eight pieces of oranges, four pieces of Roma tomatoes, twenty baby carrots, and broccoli leaves, and add water. Before blending, at the top of the blender, leave one to one and a half inches empty to leave room for blending. Blend or liquefy for five minutes. Place in the gallon container. If needed, add additional water to the gallon to make eight cups of water. (This may vary depending on the cup size of the blender.)

4. Place the top on the gallon container and shake well for a few minutes. Adding sugar is not recommended, and if on a diet, avoid using sugar. To sweeten, add no more than one-third cup of organic whole cane sugar (brown sugar). Stir and place in refrigerator until cold. For a fresh taste, drink within three to five days or store in the freezer.

Research shows, over time, this may help reduce the risk of certain forms of cancer and heart disease and may help reduce blood cholesterol.

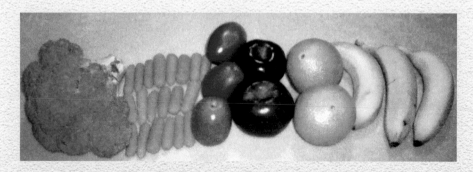

PINEAPPLE BLEND

½ pineapple
2 oranges (seedless)
2 bananas
20 baby carrots
2 cabbage leaves
7 ½ cups of water
(Remember to wash all fruits and vegetables thoroughly.)

1. Peel two bananas and cut them into three pieces each. Peel two seedless oranges and cut them into four pieces each. Remove twenty baby carrots from the bag. Break off two fresh cabbage leaves from a head of cabbage and cut each leaf into three pieces. Take one pineapple and cut it in half, remove the skin and crown and cut it into eight pieces. Place the other portion of cabbage and pineapple in the refrigerator.

2. Place in a blender six pieces of bananas, eight pieces of oranges, and twenty baby carrots, and add three to three and a half cups of water. Before blending, at the top of the blender, leave one to one and a half inches empty to leave room for blending. Blend or liquefy for five minutes. Place in the gallon container. (This may vary depending on the cup size of the blender.)

3. Place in the blender eight pieces of pineapple and six pieces of cabbage leaves and add water. Before blending, at the top of the blender, leave one to one and a half inches empty to leave room for blending. Blend or liquefy for five minutes. Place in the gallon container. If needed, add additional water to the gallon to make seven and a half cups of water. (This may vary depending on the cup size of the blender.)

4. Place the top on the gallon container and shake well for a few minutes. Adding sugar is not recommended, and if on a diet, avoid using sugar. To sweeten, add no more than one-third cup of organic whole cane sugar (brown sugar). Stir and place in refrigerator until cold. For a fresh taste, drink within three to five days or store in the freezer.

Research shows, over time, this may help protect against the risk of certain forms of cancer and promote good health.

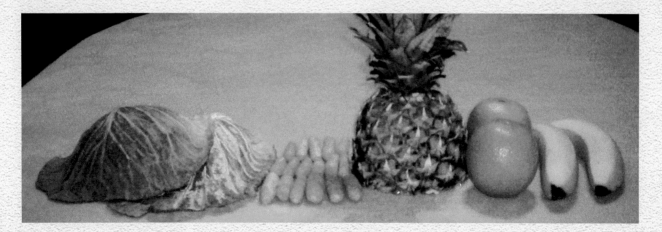

FRUITY FUN BLEND

2 apples
2 pears
2 oranges (seedless)
2 bananas
20 baby carrots
15 baby spinach leaves
8 cups of water
(Remember to wash all fruits and vegetables thoroughly.)

1. Peel two bananas and cut them into three pieces each. Peel two seedless oranges and cut them into four pieces each. Cut two apples into four pieces each and remove the seeds. Cut two pears into four pieces each and remove the stalk. Remove twenty baby carrots from the bag, and remove fifteen fresh baby spinach leaves from the bag.

2. Place in a blender three pieces of bananas, eight pieces of apples, and eight pieces of pears, and add three and a half to four cups of water. Before blending, at the top of the blender, leave one to one and a half inches empty to leave room for blending. Blend or liquefy for five minutes. Place in the gallon container. (This may vary depending on the cup size of the blender.)

3. Place in blender eight pieces of oranges, three pieces of bananas, twenty baby carrots, and fifteen baby spinach leaves, and add water. Before blending, at the top of the blender, leave one to one and a half inches empty to leave room for blending. Blend or liquefy for five minutes. Place in the gallon container. If needed, add additional water to the gallon to make eight cups of water. (This may vary depending on the cup size of the blender.)

4. Place the top on the gallon container and shake well for a few minutes. Adding sugar is not recommended, and if on a diet, avoid using sugar. To sweeten, add no more than one-third cup of organic whole cane sugar (brown sugar). Stir and place in refrigerator until cold. For a fresh taste, drink within three to five days or store in the freezer.

Research shows, over time, this may help reduce the risk of certain forms of cancer and heart disease and promote good health.

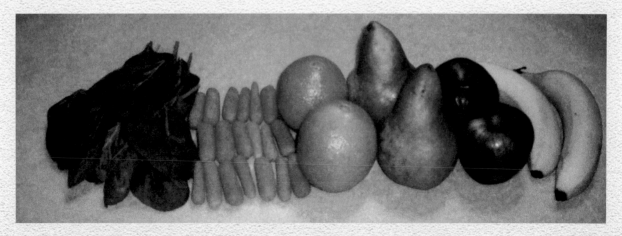

PINEAPPLE-PLUS BLEND

1 pineapple
3 bananas
3 tomatoes (Roma)
20 baby carrots
2 kale leaves
8 cups of water
(Remember to wash all fruits and vegetables thoroughly.)

1. Peel three bananas and cut them into three pieces each. Cut three Roma tomatoes into two pieces each. Remove twenty baby carrots from the bag. Cut the stems off two kale leaves and cut each leaf into three pieces. Take one pineapple, remove the skin and crown and cut them into twelve pieces.

2. Place in blender nine pieces of bananas, six pieces of Roma tomatoes, twenty baby carrots, and six pieces of kale leaves, and add three to three and a half cups of water. Before blending, at the top of the blender, leave one to one and a half inches empty to leave room for blending. Blend or liquefy for five minutes. Place in the gallon container. (This may vary depending on the cup size of the blender.)

3. Place in blender twelve pieces of pineapple, and add water. Before blending, at the top of the blender, leave one to one and a half inches empty to leave room for blending. Blend or liquefy for five minutes. Place in the gallon container. If needed, add additional water to the gallon to make eight cups of water. (This may vary depending on the cup size of the blender.)

4. Place the top on the gallon container and shake well for a few minutes. Adding sugar is not recommended, and if on a diet, avoid using sugar. To sweeten, add no more than one-third cup of organic whole cane sugar (brown sugar). Stir and place in refrigerator until cold. For a fresh taste, drink within three to five days or store in the freezer.

Research shows, over time, this may help reduce the risk of certain forms of cancer and heart disease and help support the immune system.

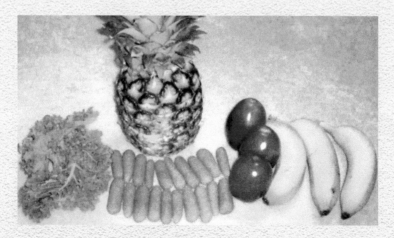

MORNING BLEND

½ honeydew
3 bananas
2 plums
2 tomatoes (Roma)
2 turnip greens (leaves)
6 to 7 cups of water
(Remember to wash all fruits and vegetables thoroughly.)

1. Peel three bananas and cut them into three pieces each. Cut two Roma tomatoes into two pieces each. Cut two plums into two pieces each and remove the seeds. Cut two turnip leaves into three pieces each. Take one honeydew and cut it in half, remove the skin, and cut it into eight pieces. Place the other portion of honeydew in the refrigerator.

2. Place in a blender eight pieces of peaches, eight pieces of oranges, and twenty baby carrots, and add four to four and a half cups of water. Before blending, at the top of the blender, leave one to one and a half inches empty to leave room for blending. Blend or liquefy for five minutes. Place in the gallon container. (This may vary depending on the cup size of the blender.)

3. Place in the blender eight pieces of cantaloupe and six pieces of turnip leaves and add water. Before blending, at the top of the blender, leave one to one and a half inches empty to leave room for blending. Blend or liquefy for five minutes. Place in the gallon container. If needed, add additional water to the gallon to make eight cups of water. (This may vary depending on the cup size of the blender.)

4. Place the top on the gallon container and shake well for a few minutes. Adding sugar is not recommended, and if on a diet, avoid using sugar. To sweeten, add no more than one-third cup of organic whole cane sugar (brown sugar). Stir and place in refrigerator until cold. For a fresh taste, drink within three to five days or store in the freezer.

Research shows, over time, this may help boost the immune system and promote good health.

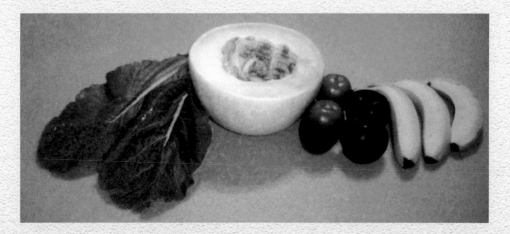

FUN BURST BLEND

3 oranges (seedless)
3 nectarines
3 peaches
3 bananas
2 turnip greens (leaves)
8 cups of water
(Remember to wash all fruits and vegetables thoroughly.)

1. Peel three bananas and cut them into three pieces each. Peel three seedless oranges and cut them into four pieces each. Cut three peaches into four pieces each and remove the seeds. Cut three nectarines into four pieces each and remove the seeds, and cut two turnip leaves into three pieces each.

2. Place in a blender nine pieces of bananas, four pieces of peaches, four pieces of seedless oranges, and six pieces of turnip leaves, and add three to three and a half cups of water. Before blending, at the top of the blender, leave one to one and a half inches empty to leave room for blending. Blend or liquefy for five minutes. Place in the gallon container. (This may vary depending on the cup size of the blender.)

3. Place in the blender twelve pieces of nectarine, eight pieces of peaches, and eight pieces of seedless oranges, and add water. Before blending, at the top of the blender, leave one to one and a half inches empty to leave room for blending. Blend or liquefy for five minutes. Place in the gallon container. If needed, add additional water to the gallon to make eight cups of water. (This may vary depending on the cup size of the blender.)

4. Place the top on the gallon container and shake well for a few minutes. Adding sugar is not recommended, and if on a diet, avoid using sugar. To sweeten, add no more than one-third cup of organic whole cane sugar (brown sugar). Stir and place in refrigerator until cold. For a fresh taste, drink within three to five days or store in the freezer.

Research shows, over time, this may help reduce the risk of certain forms of cancer and promote good health.

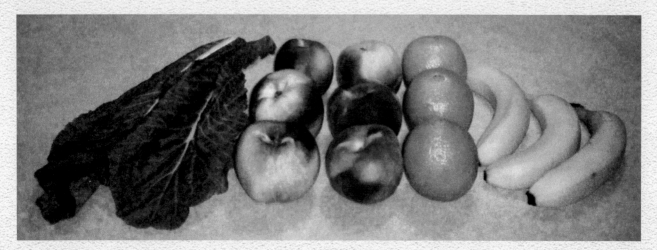

MIDDAY BLEND

1 cantaloupe
10 strawberries
2 bananas
3 tomatoes (Roma)
3 mustard greens (leaves)
7 to 8 cups of water
(Remember to wash all fruits and vegetables thoroughly.)

1. Peel two bananas and cut them into three pieces each. Cut three Roma tomatoes into two pieces each. Remove the green leaves off the top of ten strawberries and cut each strawberry into two pieces. Cut three mustard leaves into three pieces each. Take one cantaloupe, remove the skin, and cut it into sixteen pieces.

2. Place in a blender six pieces of cantaloupe, twenty pieces of strawberries, and three pieces of mustard leaves, and add two and a half to three cups of water. Before blending, at the top of the blender, leave one to one and a half inches empty to leave room for blending. Blend or liquefy for five minutes. Place in the gallon container. (This may vary depending on the cup size of the blender.)

3. Place in the blender four pieces of cantaloupe, six pieces of Roma tomatoes, and six pieces of mustard leaves, and add water. Before blending, at the top of the blender, leave one to one and a half inches empty to leave room for blending. Blend or liquefy for five minutes. Place in the gallon container. (This may vary depending on the cup size of the blender.)

4. Place in the blender six pieces of bananas and six pieces of cantaloupe and add water. Before blending, at the top of the blender, leave one to one and a half inches empty to leave room for blending. Blend or liquefy for five minutes. Place in the gallon container. If needed, add additional water to the gallon to make seven to eight cups of water. (This may vary depending on the cup size of the blender.)

5. Place the top on the gallon container and shake well for a few minutes. Adding sugar is not recommended, and if on a diet, avoid using sugar. To sweeten, add no more than one-third cup of organic whole cane sugar (brown sugar). Stir and place in refrigerator until cold. For a fresh taste, drink within three to five days or store in the freezer.

Research shows, over time, this may help reduce the risk of certain forms of cancer and support the immune system.

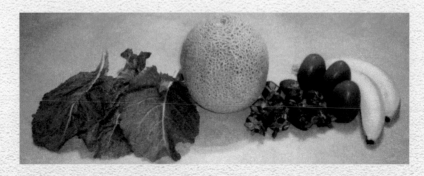

DAYBREAK BLEND

1 cantaloupe
3 bananas
1 grapefruit
20 baby carrots
1 kale leaf
9 cups of water
(Remember to wash all fruits and vegetables thoroughly.)

1. Peel three bananas and cut them into three pieces each. Peel one grapefruit and cut it into six pieces. Remove twenty baby carrots from the bag. Cut one kale leaf into three pieces. Take one cantaloupe, remove the skin, and cut it into sixteen pieces.

2. Place in a blender nine pieces of bananas, three pieces of kale leaves, and three pieces of cantaloupe, and add two and a half to three cups of water. Before blending, at the top of the blender, leave one to one and a half inches empty to leave room for blending. Blend or liquefy for five minutes. Place in the gallon container. (This may vary depending on the cup size of the blender.)

3. Place in the blender six pieces of grapefruit, twenty baby carrots, and three pieces of cantaloupe, and add two and a half to three cups of water. Before blending, at the top of the blender, leave one to one and a half inches empty to leave room for blending. Blend or liquefy for five minutes. Place in the gallon container. (This may vary depending on the cup size of the blender.)

4. Place in the blender ten pieces of cantaloupe and add water. Before blending, at the top of the blender, leave one to one and a half inches empty to leave room for blending. Blend or liquefy for five minutes. Place in the gallon container. If needed, add additional water to the gallon to make nine cups of water. (This may vary depending on the cup size of the blender.)

5. Place the top on the gallon container and shake well for a few minutes. Adding sugar is not recommended, and if on a diet, avoid using sugar. To sweeten, add no more than one-third cup of organic whole cane sugar (brown sugar). Stir and place in refrigerator until cold. For a fresh taste, drink within three to five days or store in the freezer.

Research shows, over time, this may help reduce the risk of certain forms of cancer and heart disease and support the immune system.

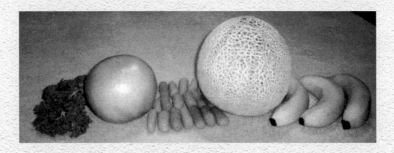

MIDAFTERNOON BLEND

1/3 watermelon (seedless)
2 bananas
2 peaches
20 baby carrots
3 turnip greens (leaves)
8 cups of water
(Remember to wash all fruits and vegetables thoroughly.)

1. Peel two bananas and cut them into three pieces each. Cut two peaches into four pieces each and remove the seeds. Remove twenty baby carrots from the bag. Cut three turnip leaves into three pieces each. Cut one-third of a watermelon and cut the portion into twelve pieces. Place the other portion of watermelon in the refrigerator.

2. Place in a blender six pieces of bananas, four pieces of peaches, twenty baby carrots, and six pieces of turnip leaves, and add three and a half to four cups of water. Before blending, at the top of the blender, leave one to one and a half inches empty to leave room for blending. Blend or liquefy for five minutes. Place in the gallon container. (This may vary depending on the cup size of the blender.)

3. Place in the blender five pieces of watermelon and four pieces of peaches and add water. Before blending, at the top of the blender, leave one to one and a half inches empty to leave room for blending. Blend or liquefy for five minutes. Place in the gallon container. (This may vary depending on the cup size of the blender.)

4. Place in the blender seven pieces of watermelon and three pieces of turnip leaves and add water. Before blending, at the top of the blender, leave one to one and a half inches empty to leave room for blending. If needed, add additional water to the gallon to make eight cups of water. (This may vary depending on the cup size of the blender.)

5. Place the top on the gallon container and shake well for a few minutes. Adding sugar is not recommended, and if on a diet, avoid using sugar. To sweeten, add no more than one-third cup of organic whole cane sugar (brown sugar). Stir and place in refrigerator until cold. For a fresh taste, drink within three to five days or store in the freezer.

Research shows, over time, this may help reduce the risk of certain forms of cancer and promote good health.

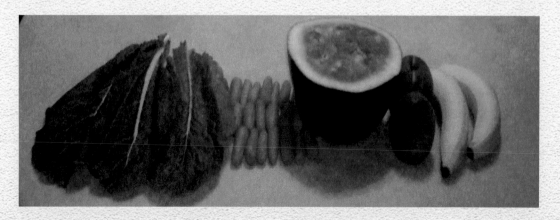

SUNSET BLEND

½ honeydew
3 bananas
2 oranges (seedless)
2 tomatoes (Roma)
2 mustard greens (leaves)
6 to 7 cups of water
(Remember to wash all fruits and vegetables thoroughly.)

1. Peel three bananas and cut them into three pieces each. Cut two Roma tomatoes into two pieces each. Peel two seedless oranges and cut them into four pieces each. Cut two mustard leaves into three pieces each. Take one honeydew and cut it in half. Remove the skin and cut it into ten pieces. Place the other portion of honeydew in the refrigerator.

2. Place in blender nine pieces of bananas, eight pieces of oranges, and four pieces of Roma tomatoes, and add three to three and a half cups of water. Before blending, at the top of the blender, leave one to one and a half inches empty to leave room for blending. Blend or liquefy for five minutes. Place in the gallon container. (This may vary depending on the cup size of the blender.)

3. Place in blender ten pieces of honeydew and six pieces of mustard leaves and add water. Before blending, at the top of the blender, leave one to one and a half inches empty to leave room for blending. Blend or liquefy for five minutes. Place in the gallon container. If needed, add additional water to the gallon to make six to seven cups of water. (This may vary depending on the cup size of the blender.)

4. Place the top on the gallon container and shake well for a few minutes. Adding sugar is not recommended, and if on a diet, avoid using sugar. To sweeten, add no more than one-third cup of organic whole cane sugar (brown sugar). Stir and place in refrigerator until cold. For a fresh taste, drink within three to five days or store in the freezer.

Research shows, over time, this may help support the immune system.

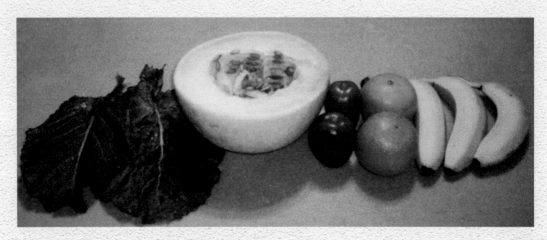

TASTY BLEND

2 bananas
2 apples
2 oranges (seedless)
3 tomatoes (Roma)
20 baby carrots
3 collard greens (leaves)
8 cups of water
(Remember to wash all fruits and vegetables thoroughly.)

1. Peel two bananas and cut them into three pieces each. Cut two apples into four pieces each and remove the seeds. Peel two seedless oranges and cut them into four pieces each. Cut three Roma tomatoes into two pieces each, remove twenty baby carrots from the bag, and cut three collard leaves into three pieces each.

2. Place in a blender six pieces of bananas, twenty baby carrots, and nine pieces of collard leaves, and add three and a half to four cups of water. Before blending, at the top of the blender, leave one to one and a half inches empty to leave room for blending. Blend or liquefy for five minutes. Place in the gallon container. (This may vary depending on the cup size of the blender.)

3. Place in the blender eight pieces of apples, eight pieces of oranges, and six pieces of Roma tomatoes, and add water. Before blending, at the top of the blender, leave one to one and a half inches empty to leave room for blending. Blend or liquefy for five minutes. Place in the gallon container. If needed, add additional water to the gallon to make eight cups of water. (This may vary depending on the cup size of the blender.)

4. Place the top on the gallon container and shake well for a few minutes. Adding sugar is not recommended, and if on a diet, avoid using sugar. To sweeten, add no more than one-third cup of organic whole cane sugar (brown sugar). Stir and place in refrigerator until cold. For a fresh taste, drink within three to five days or store in the freezer.

Research shows, over time, this may help reduce the risk of certain forms of cancer and reduce blood cholesterol.

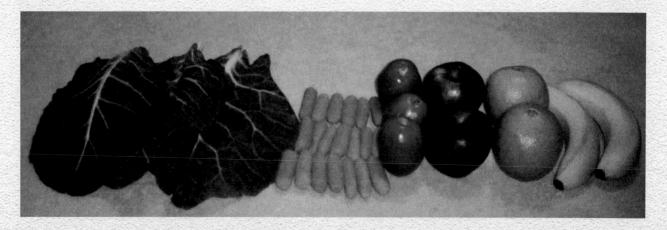

MELON BLEND

1/3 watermelon (seedless)
2 oranges (seedless)
2 bananas
2 tomatoes (Roma)
3 mustard greens (leaves)
7 cups of water
(Remember to wash all fruits and vegetables thoroughly.)

1. Peel two bananas and cut them into three pieces each. Peel two seedless oranges and cut them into four pieces each. Cut two Roma tomatoes into two pieces each. Cut three mustard leaves into three pieces each. Cut one-third of a watermelon and cut the portion into twelve pieces. Place the other portion of watermelon in the refrigerator.

2. Place in a blender six pieces of bananas, eight pieces of oranges, and nine pieces of mustard leaves, and add two and a half to three cups of water. Before blending, at the top of the blender, leave one to one and a half inches empty to leave room for blending. Blend or liquefy for five minutes. Place in the gallon container. (This may vary depending on the cup size of the blender.)

3. Place in the blender four pieces of Roma tomatoes and four pieces of watermelon and add water. Before blending, at the top of the blender, leave one to one and a half inches empty to leave room for blending. Place in the gallon container. (This may vary depending on the cup size of the blender.)

4. Place in blender eight pieces of watermelon and add water. Before blending, at the top of the blender, leave one to one and a half inches empty to leave room for blending. Blend or liquefy for five minutes. Place in the gallon container. If needed, add additional water to the gallon to make seven cups of water. (This may vary depending on the cup size of the blender.)

5. Place the top on the gallon container and shake well for a few minutes. Adding sugar is not recommended, and if on a diet, avoid using sugar. To sweeten, add no more than one-third cup of organic whole cane sugar (brown sugar). Stir and place in refrigerator until cold. For a fresh taste, drink within three to five days or store in the freezer.

Research shows, over time, this may help reduce the risk of certain forms of cancer and support the immune system.

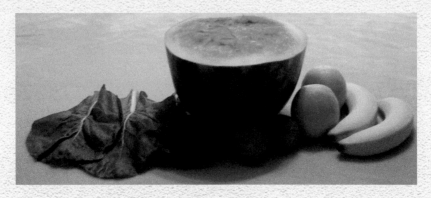

GRAPEFRUIT BLEND

1 grapefruit (seedless)
2 apples
3 bananas
2 tomatoes (Roma)
1 broccoli bunch
7 to 8 cups of water
(Remember to wash all fruits and vegetables thoroughly.)

1. Peel three bananas and cut them into three pieces each. Cut two apples into four pieces each and remove the seeds. Peel one grapefruit (seedless) and cut it into four pieces. Cut two Roma tomatoes into two pieces each. Take one broccoli bunch and cut off the stem and chop the leaves into pieces.

2. Place in a blender nine pieces of bananas, four pieces of apples, and four pieces of Roma tomatoes, and add three to three and a half cups of water. Before blending, at the top of the blender, leave one to one and a half inches empty to leave room for blending. Blend or liquefy for five minutes. Place in the gallon container. (This may vary depending on the cup size of the blender.)

3. Place in the blender four pieces of apples, four pieces of grapefruit, and broccoli leaves, and add water. Before blending, at the top of the blender, leave one to one and a half inches empty to leave room for blending. Blend or liquefy for five minutes. Place in the gallon container. If needed, add additional water to the gallon to make seven to eight cups of water. (This may vary depending on the cup size of the blender.)

4. Place the top on the gallon container and shake well for a few minutes. Adding sugar is not recommended, and if on a diet, avoid using sugar. To sweeten, add no more than one-third cup of organic whole cane sugar (brown sugar). Stir and place in refrigerator until cold. For a fresh taste, drink within three to five days or store in the freezer.

Research shows, over time, this may help reduce blood cholesterol and promote good health.

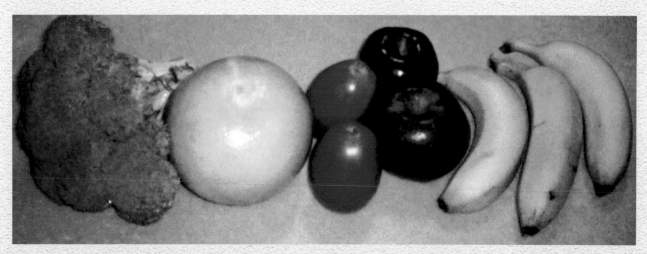

FRUIT TASTY BLEND

2 bananas
2 apples
2 oranges (seedless)
2 tomatoes (Roma)
20 baby carrots
3 collard greens (leaves)
8 cups of water
(Remember to wash all fruits and vegetables thoroughly.)

1. Peel two bananas and cut them into three pieces each. Cut two apples into four pieces each and remove the seeds. Peel two seedless oranges and cut them into four pieces each. Cut two Roma tomatoes into two pieces each, remove twenty baby carrots from the bag, and cut three collard leaves into three pieces each.

2. Place in a blender six pieces of bananas, twenty baby carrots, and nine pieces of collard leaves, and add three and a half to four cups of water. Before blending, at the top of the blender, leave one to one and a half inches empty to leave room for blending. Blend or liquefy for five minutes. Place in the gallon container. (This may vary depending on the cup size of the blender.)

3. Place in the blender eight pieces of apples, eight pieces of oranges, and four pieces of Roma tomatoes, and add water. Before blending, at the top of the blender, leave one to one and a half inches empty to leave room for blending. Blend or liquefy for five minutes. Place in the gallon container. If needed, add additional water to the gallon to make eight cups of water. (This may vary depending on the cup size of the blender.)

4. Place the top on the gallon container and shake well for a few minutes. Adding sugar is not recommended, and if on a diet, avoid using sugar. To sweeten, add no more than one-third cup of organic whole cane sugar (brown sugar). Stir and place in refrigerator until cold. For a fresh taste, drink within three to five days or store in the freezer.

Research shows, over time, this may help reduce the risk of certain forms of cancer and may help reduce blood cholesterol.

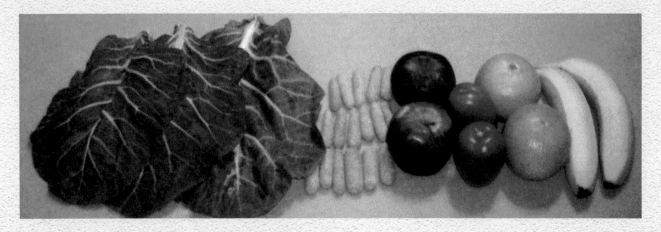

COLLARD BLEND

2 peaches
1 apple
2 oranges (seedless)
2 bananas
3 collard greens (leaves)
20 baby carrots
9 cups of water
(Remember to wash all fruits and vegetables thoroughly.)

1. Peel two bananas and cut them into three pieces each. Cut one apple into four pieces each and remove the seeds. Peel two seedless oranges and cut them into four pieces each. Cut two peaches into four pieces each and remove the seeds. Remove twenty baby carrots from the bag, and cut three collard leaves into three pieces each.

2. Place in a blender four pieces of apples, four pieces of peaches, twenty baby carrots, and nine pieces of collard leaves, and add three to three and a half cups of water. Before blending, at the top of the blender, leave one to one and a half inches empty to leave room for blending. Blend or liquefy for five minutes. Place in the gallon container. (This may vary depending on the cup size of the blender.)

3. Place in the blender eight pieces of oranges, four pieces of peaches, and six pieces of bananas, and add water. Before blending, at the top of the blender, leave one to one and a half inches empty to leave room for blending. Blend or liquefy for five minutes. Place in the gallon container. If needed, add additional water to the gallon to make nine cups of water. (This may vary depending on the cup size of the blender.)

4. Place the top of the gallon container and shake well for a few minutes. Adding sugar is not recommended, and if on a diet, avoid using sugar. To sweeten, add no more than one-third cup of organic whole cane sugar (brown sugar). Stir and place in refrigerator until cold. For a fresh taste, drink within three to five days or store in the freezer.

Research shows, over time, this may help reduce the risk of certain forms of heart disease and reduce blood cholesterol.

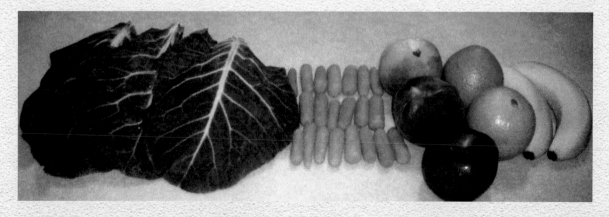

FRUITY-PLUS BLEND

3 oranges (seedless)
3 apples
3 bananas
20 baby carrots
2 collard greens (leaves)
8 cups of water
(Remember to wash all fruits and vegetables thoroughly.)

1. Peel three bananas and cut them into three pieces each. Cut three apples into four pieces each and remove the seeds. Peel three seedless oranges and cut them into four pieces each, remove twenty baby carrots from the bag, and cut two collard leaves into three pieces each.

2. Place in a blender twelve pieces of oranges, twenty baby carrots, and six pieces of collard leaves, and add three to three and a half cups of water. Before blending, at the top of the blender, leave one to one and a half inches empty to leave room for blending. Blend or liquefy for five minutes. Place in the gallon container. (This may vary depending on the cup size of the blender.)

3. Place in the blender twelve pieces of apples and nine pieces of bananas and add water. Before blending, at the top of the blender, leave one to one and a half inches empty to leave room for blending. Blend or liquefy for five minutes. Place in the gallon container. If needed, add additional water to the gallon to make eight cups of water. (This may vary depending on the cup size of the blender.)

4. Place the top of the gallon container and shake well for a few minutes. Adding sugar is not recommended, and if on a diet, avoid using sugar. To sweeten, add no more than one-third cup of organic whole cane sugar (brown sugar). Stir and place in refrigerator until cold. For a fresh taste, drink within three to five days or store in the freezer.

Research shows, over time, this may help reduce blood cholesterol and promote good health.

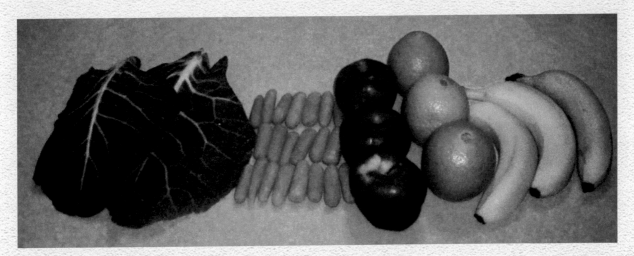

MIDEVENING BLEND

3 oranges (seedless)
2 plums
2 bananas
3 tomatoes (Roma)
2 collard greens (leaves)
8 cups water
(Remember to wash all fruits and vegetables thoroughly.)

1. Peel two bananas and cut them into three pieces each. Cut two plums into four pieces each and remove the seeds. Peel three seedless oranges and cut them into four pieces each. Cut three Roma tomatoes into two pieces each, and cut two collard leaves into three pieces each.

2. Place in a blender six pieces of bananas, six pieces of Roma tomatoes, and six pieces of collard leaves, and add three to three and a half cups of water. Before blending, at the top of the blender, leave one to one and a half inches empty to leave room for blending. Blend or liquefy for five minutes. Place in the gallon container. (This may vary depending on the cup size of the blender.)

3. Place in the blender eight pieces of plums and twelve pieces of oranges and add water. Before blending, at the top of the blender, leave one to one and a half inches empty to leave room for blending. Blend or liquefy for five minutes. Place in the gallon container. If needed, add additional water to the gallon to make eight cups of water. (This may vary depending on the cup size of the blender.)

4. Place the top on the gallon container and shake well for a few minutes. Adding sugar is not recommended, and if on a diet, avoid using sugar. To sweeten, add no more than one-third cup of organic whole cane sugar (brown sugar). Stir and place in refrigerator until cold. For a fresh taste, drink within three to five days or store in the freezer.

Research shows, over time, this may help promote good health and support the immune system.

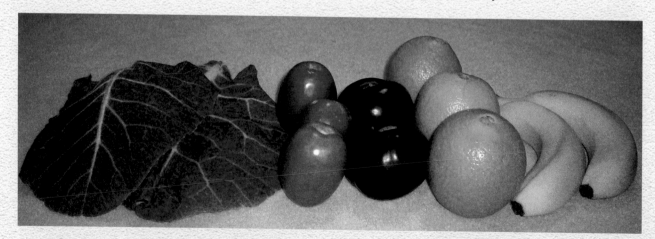

VEGETABLE-PLUS BLEND

3 bananas
3 oranges (seedless)
2 apples
2 collard greens (leaves)
20 baby spinach leaves
8 cups of water
(Remember to wash all fruits and vegetables thoroughly.)

1. Peel three bananas and cut them into three pieces each. Cut two apples into four pieces each and remove the seeds. Peel three seedless oranges and cut them into four pieces each, remove twenty fresh baby spinach leaves from the bag, and cut two collard leaves into three pieces each.

2. Place in a blender three pieces of bananas, eight pieces of oranges, twenty baby spinach, and six pieces of collard leaves, and add three and a half to four cups of water. Before blending, at the top of the blender, leave one to one and a half inches empty to leave room for blending. Blend or liquefy for five minutes. Place in the gallon container. (This may vary depending on the cup size of the blender.)

3. Place in the blender six pieces of bananas, four pieces of oranges, and eight pieces of apples, and add water. Before blending, at the top of the blender, leave one to one and a half inches empty to leave room for blending. Blend or liquefy for five minutes. Place in the gallon container. If needed, add additional water to the gallon to make eight cups of water. (This may vary depending on the cup size of the blender.)

4. Place the top on the gallon container and shake well for a few minutes. Adding sugar is not recommended, and if on a diet, avoid using sugar. To sweeten, add no more than one-third cup of organic whole cane sugar (brown sugar). Stir and place in refrigerator until cold. For a fresh taste, drink within three to five days or store in the freezer.

Research shows, over time, this may help reduce blood cholesterol and promote good health.

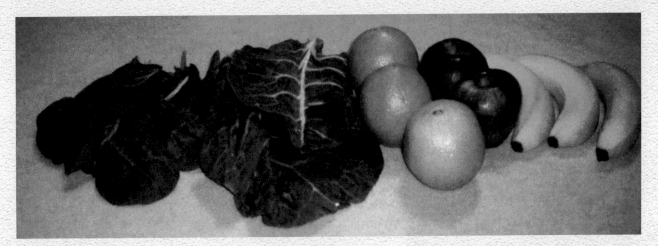

CANTALOUPE BLEND

1 cantaloupe
2 bananas
2 peaches
20 baby carrots
2 cabbage leaves
7 cups of water
(Remember to wash all fruits and vegetables thoroughly.)

1. Peel two bananas and cut them into three pieces each. Cut two peaches into four pieces each and remove the seeds. Remove twenty baby carrots from the bag. Break off two fresh cabbage leaves from a head of cabbage and cut each leaf into three pieces. Take one cantaloupe and remove the skin and cut it into sixteen pieces. Place the other portion of the cabbage in the refrigerator.

2. Place in a blender eight pieces of cantaloupe, six pieces of cabbage leaves, and three pieces of bananas, and add two and a half to three cups of water. Before blending, at the top of the blender, leave one to one and a half inches empty to leave room for blending. Blend or liquefy for five minutes. Place in the gallon container. (This may vary depending on the cup size of the blender.)

3. Place in the blender four pieces of cantaloupe, eight pieces of peaches, and three pieces of bananas, and add water. Before blending, at the top of the blender, leave one to one and a half inches empty to leave room for blending. Blend or liquefy for five minutes. Place in the gallon container. (This may vary depending on the cup size of the blender.)

4. Place in the blender four pieces of cantaloupe and twenty baby carrots, and add water. Before blending, at the top of the blender, leave one to one and a half inches empty to leave room for blending. Blend or liquefy for five minutes. Place in the gallon container. If needed, add additional water to the gallon to make seven cups of water. (This may vary depending on the cup size of the blender.)

5. Place the top on the gallon container and shake well for a few minutes. Adding sugar is not recommended, and if on a diet avoid, using sugar. To sweeten, add no more than one-third cup of organic whole cane sugar (brown sugar). Stir and place in refrigerator until cold. For a fresh taste, drink within three to five days or store in the freezer.

Research shows, over time, this may help support the immune system and promote good health.

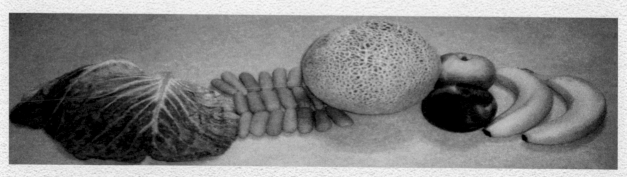

WATERMELON BLEND

1/3 watermelon (seedless)
15 strawberries
2 bananas
20 baby spinach leaves
10 baby carrots
6 ½ cups of water
(Remember to wash all fruits and vegetables thoroughly.)

1. Peel two bananas and cut them into three pieces each. Remove the green leaves off the top of the fifteen strawberries and cut each strawberry into two pieces. Remove ten baby carrots from the bag, and remove twenty fresh baby spinach leaves from the bag. Cut one-third of a watermelon and cut the portion into twelve pieces. Place the other portion of watermelon in the refrigerator.

2. Place in a blender thirty pieces of strawberries, ten baby carrots, and six pieces of bananas, and add two to two and a half cups of water. Before blending, at the top of the blender, leave one to one and a half inches empty to leave room for blending. Blend or liquefy for five minutes. Place in the gallon container. (This may vary depending on the cup size of the blender.)

3. Place in the blender six pieces of watermelon and twenty baby spinach leaves and add water. Before blending, at the top of the blender, leave one to one and a half inches empty to leave room for blending. Blend of liquefy for five minutes. Place in the gallon container. (This may vary depending on the cup size of the blender.)

4. Place in the blender six pieces of watermelon and add water. Before blending, at the top of the blender, leave one to one and a half inches empty to leave room for blending. Blend or liquefy for five minutes. Place in the gallon container. If needed, add additional water to the gallon to make six and a half cups of water. (This may vary depending on the cup size of the blender.)

5. Place the top on the gallon container and shake well for a few minutes. Adding sugar is not recommended, and if on a diet, avoid using sugar. To sweeten, add no more than one-third cup of organic whole cane sugar (brown sugar). Place in refrigerator until cold. For a fresh taste, drink within three to five days or store in the freezer.

Research shows, over time, this may help support the immune system and promote good health.

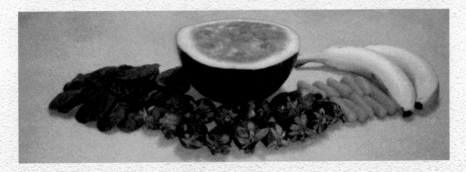

TURNIP BLEND

1 squash (yellow)
3 plums
3 oranges (seedless)
2 tomatoes (Roma)
4 turnip greens (leaves)
10 cups of water
(Remember to wash all fruits and vegetables thoroughly.)

1. Cut one squash into four pieces each. Cut three plums into four pieces each and remove the seeds. Peel three seedless oranges and cut them into four pieces each. Cut two Roma tomatoes into two pieces each. Cut four turnip leaves into three pieces each.

2. Place in a blender four pieces of squash, twelve pieces of oranges, and six pieces of turnip leaves, and add three to three and a half cups of water. Before blending, at the top of the blender, leave one to one and a half inches empty to leave room for blending. Blend or liquefy for five minutes. Place in the gallon container. (This may vary depending on the cup size of the blender.)

3. Place in the blender twelve pieces of plums, four pieces of tomatoes, and six pieces of turnip leaves and add water. Before blending, at the top of the blender, leave one to one and a half inches empty to leave room for blending. Blend or liquefy for five minutes. Place in the gallon container. If needed, add additional water to the gallon to make ten cups of water. (This may vary depending on the cup size of the blender.)

4. Place the top on the gallon container and shake well for a few minutes. Adding sugar is not recommended, and if on a diet, avoid using sugar. To sweeten, add no more than one-half cup of organic whole cane sugar (brown sugar). Stir and place in refrigerator until cold. For a fresh taste, drink within three to five days or store in the freezer.

Research shows, over time, this may help support the immune system and promote good health.

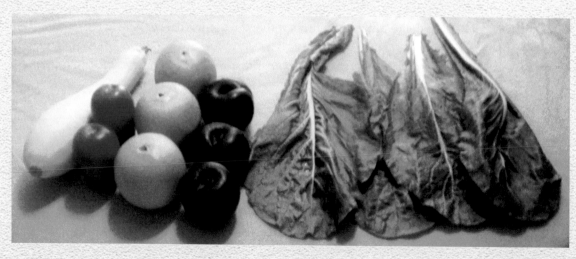

Printed in the United States
by Baker & Taylor Publisher Services